The Psych Ward:
Losing To Bipolar Disorder And Starting Life Again

Sylvia Meier

Limits of Liability / Disclaimer of Warranty:

The authors of this information and the accompanying materials have used their best efforts in preparing this course. The authors make no representation or warranties with respect to the accuracy, applicability, fitness, or completeness of the contents of this course. They disclaim any warranties (expressed or implied), merchantability, or fitness for any particular purpose. The authors shall in no event be held liable for any loss or other damages, including but not limited to special, incidental, consequential, or other damages.

DEDICATION

To those who have walked the four walls with hospital pants and shirt on, no shoes, and for sure no belt, this book is for you.

For those who have showered in stalls that have no hooks, or curtains, this book is for you.

To those who have slept in a room with a stranger who made you feel a little less crazy, this book is for you.

To those of you who learned that those four walls are not a prison but a new start, this book is for you.

For all those who love and visit those four walls to see the people you love, this book is for you.

For those of you who battle stigma and fight the looks that you ever spent time in a psych ward, this book is definitely for you.

To my family, to my children, to those in my world who came within those 4 walls to see me, I love you, and this book is for you.

"Nothing in the universe can stop you from letting go and starting over."

- Guy Finley

Sylvia Meier

CONTENTS

Introduction:

Stigma. That's what I think of when I think of mental illness. Still. Even with all my own battles, fighting my own demons, stigma s are the first thing that comes to mind.

With the psych ward it was no different. I had so many ideas of what it was like, the stigma attached to saying, yeah, I went a little crazy and spent some time in the psych ward.

It simply couldn't be left that it is a place with four walls.

It simply cannot be left that it is a place where people so at the end of their ropes go to get help.

It couldn't be left that it is a place that offers hope to the hopeless.

No.

It has to carry that painful, I've spent time in the psych ward stigma.

Or does it?

I'm not proud by any means to tell this story. But I'm not to proud to not tell this story.

If this helps one person change their perspective. If it helps a single person not reach for the knife, the noose, the bottle. If it helps a single soul, it was worth the stigma I will carry for my own time spent locked away in 4 bare white walls, with no belt, and no shoes, in a place I will forever remember. In a place called the Psych ward.

Chapter 1
The Lead Up

I've been asked in the year since my attempt on my own life if I had planned to do it. Like it was some big thing on a to do list. Like it was just another check box for the day.

Feed cats. Check.

Do laundry. Check.

Do dishes. Check.

Take my own life.

It wasn't planned.

It was the furthest thing from planned.

It was one of those moments where the dark dog bit into me. Swallowed me whole, and lead me to swallowing that handful of pills.

I could never take my own life by slicing my wrists. Who would have to clean up the blood? What stains would it leave where I died? Blood is so tough to get out of things. I hate the sight of blood.

Nope, not even the biting depression could make me die that way.

Hanging. No way. Too complicated. Too hard to make a noose. Did I even know how to make a noose? I wasn't going to sit down and Google how to make a noose. Couldn't be death by hanging.

In a single moment of darkness, my mind raced. There had

to be a way out. There had to be an easy way to do this, without mess, without difficulties.

Suffocation? You cannot suffocate yourself. Or at least I don't think you can. Something about stopping it because you would lose grip on whatever you were suffocating yourself with when you lost consciousness. Suffocating just wouldn't do.

Then the dog barked loudly in my mind. Left my soul ringing, writhing with the answer.

Pills.

Pills.

Pills.

I had medication that was to help me keep my sanity.

I had a purse full of a medical cocktail that could, if taken in large enough doses kill an elephant. And I was anything but an elephant.

I was a tiny, lost soul.

Pills it would be.

I don't really know what pushed me to that ledge. I know the fight that led me to it, but not what really allowed me to get to such a far gone state.

I don't really know how I could let that dog of depression, mania or whatever it was bite so deep. Perhaps it had nothing to do with my illness and more to do with the place in which I was in my life, the desperate situation I had found myself immersed in. I really don't to this day understand it. Except for the desperation. Except for wanting, begging for the escape from my reality, the escape from that life. That place in my life.

The night before had been amazing.

My girl, my beautiful girl had swept me off my feet. A romantic dinner. A night of holding her in my arms. The sweet embrace of love. The sweet embrace of something I wanted to feel everyday. The love I wanted to wrap myself into each night.

The night before had taken my breath away and left a smile on my heart and soul.

She once again showed me what it felt like to be loved by someone, to be connected to someone, to belong.

How did he get me so quickly, so badly, so deeply? How could he so quickly, so easily rob me of my joy, my happiness? Why couldn't I just leave?

But I digress.

However he bit into me, he had me entwined and snarled between his teeth. I had been chewed up, destroyed and spit out. My mind, heart and soul were tattered remnants on the floor.

Pills it would be.

I remember shaking as I poured them into my hand. I remember wondering how it would feel when they kicked in and took my life.

I recall wondering if it was really enough.

I recall wondering if I would be found and my body taken away before the kids got home from school.

They didn't need to see their mother's dead body. Losing me would be enough.

And in one large handful the pills went in my mouth and down my throat.

Silence.

Silence.

The front door opening.

The sound of my daughter.

Oh my gawd what am I doing.

Fingers down my throat, forcing with all my might.

Get the pills out. Get them out.

I'm not ready to die. This is not what I want.

911.

Please help.

Head on the cold, hard floor. 911. Please, please help.

I need help.

I need help.

Trying to vomit more.

Please 911 I need help as the phone drops to the floor.

Commotion around me. Swirling world.

Shit. I was too late. I was too late. I didn't really want to die.

As the dog released it's deathly bite, I realize, I don't want to die.

I remember the ambulance.

I remember the bald paramedic.

I remember our conversation.

I recall his look.

I recall him actually caring if I lived or died.

I recalled my children. I recalled my girlfriend. I recalled all those people in my life I may have lost.

I recall simply needing help and to get out of my current life so badly, so bad that my heart was broken, my soul was lost, and my mind grasped in some other reality, that for that moment I forgot all the things I had to live for in my life.

So now you know the lead-up. What follows is my 5 days in the psych ward, and learning what I really had to live for, and what I was truly fighting against.

Even as I write this the tears streak my face. I cannot imagine anyone, let alone myself in such a deep, dark place.

I cannot imagine truly what was going through my mind, and what really was the lead-up to my struggle for my own life, my struggle to keep the blood flowing through my veins, the struggle to keep living.

If you've never been there. Please don't judge.

It's a dark, ungodly, unforgiving place.

And once you've been there. To that point. Your soul is marred. Forever marked.

I will forever remember that I was in such a bad state of mind and body, that I wanted it over, all of it over, for good, but by the grace of an Angel, (take that as you will for my daughter, the one who opened that front door, her name is Angel) survived that seductress embrace of death and wanting so deeply to die.

"Life begins on the other side of despair"

    - Jean-Paul Sartre

Chapter 2:

The Entrance

Despair is the price one pays for setting oneself an impossible aim. It is, one is told, the unforgivable sin, but it is a sin the corrupt or evil man never practices. He always has hope. He never reaches the freezing-point of knowing absolute failure. Only the man of goodwill carries always in his heart this capacity for damnation.

– Greene, Graham

I was brought in by ambulance, and made to sit for well over an hour with the paramedic who made sure that I knew for no reason should I ever feel so down again. I had so much to live for and he knew one day I would tell my story. If I knew his name, or could reach out to him, I would give him the very first printed copy of this story.

I had downed lithium, that was the most concerning factor. Lithium overdose can kill, and can cause the most awful side effects on your internal organs. It can cause your body to do all sort of bad shit. I guess I hadn't thought about that when I tried to rob myself of life. The consequential effects of not completely doing it, or not completing the task.

Black, awful, horrible charcoal was forced down my throat, until I couldn't take it anymore. The most awful chalkiest, most utterly disgusting liquid that has ever passed my lips. It was to absorb anything that made it through my vomiting episodes. It was to ensure that any poison left in my body was taken away. And away it was taken in the worst possible way.

Your body cannot digest charcoal. It simply binds to everything as it goes through your system and sweeps it all out in one quick awful process. I don't know what was worse, it going in, or it coming out. Either way it was one of the very worst parts of all of it.

Questions, questions, so many questions.

Was it planned? How many times did I have to say no before someone would listen and believe it.

Why? Why would someone so young want to die? What was so bad that I wanted to end it all?

What made me stop?

Was this the first attempt?

Did I have other plans?

And on and on the questions fired, from one doctor to the next.

Tears streamed my face when I finally collapsed in the bed and realized I never wanted to die, I had simply given up on living.

That was the start of a new day and a new life for me.

If life was so very bad that I could not live it anymore, I should've either finished what I started or I would have to change my life. Little did I know how much my life would change.

From emergency once I was considered medically stable I was moved to the emergency psych area.

Armed guards stood outside the door.

A bed made right into the floor stood in the center of the room. Thin, almost paper like blankets lay on it.

Video cameras behind unbreakable glass watched my every move.

A window in the door so they could watch me.

No bathroom, no windows, nothing. Simply 4 empty, dismal walls staring back at me.

And again I broke. I broke down harder than ever this time. What the hell had I done? What the hell had I done? What was going to happen to me now? Would they lock me up and throw away the key? Would I ever see outside these four awful walls again.

Then in come the doctors. More questions. The same questions asked ten different ways. They were looking to see if what I was saying was really the truth.

I was to be moved.

I was going to the third floor.

I was going to the psych ward. Not the permanent forever one, simply short term stay, at least till they figured out where and what to do with me from there.

It was a very terrifying experience.

One I will never forget.

And I had yet to even step foot into the actual short term

psych ward. That scary place of horror movies. That place where drooling patients, shuffle around in slippers in every other movie.

I was glad to be alive, but scared of what the next step would be.

Chapter 3:

4 White Walls

"No more regrets, no more tears, no more broken hearts, no more fears, I'm starting over even if that means from here."

- Akila Sultana

The moment they moved me I began to wonder what had I gotten myself into.

My stuff was all taken away and kept locked away.

A girl was screaming and losing her mind right as I came onto the unit. She was screaming like an out of control crazy woman (which I found humorous given where I, myself was.)

I was quickly whisked into a room all by myself while the nursing staff restrained her and moved her out of the unit.

I was then told to come out of the room and sit in a chair in the middle of the area and wait.

At this point I finally get a chance to look around.

These were to be my four white walls for who knows how long. At least there was a panaramic view of the industrial area behind the hospital. Cause that wasn't depressing.

It started to hit me.

This was the hospital I had given birth to all five children in. This is where I had brought them all into the world. And here I was at the end of my world. Lost and living in my bipolar world.

After what seemed like forever I was taken into a room to fill out paperwork.

They needed to know about all my piercings, all my tattoos (I had a fresh one on my shoulder that had been done just over 24 hours prior...) We went through what the routine and expectations were to be while I was in these 4 white walls.

And then that was it.

I was released to my room.

Un-medicated. I was to remain un-medicated, untreated for my bipolar disorder until I saw a psychiatrist, sometime the next day. What a fun experience this was to be.

It was rough at the start. I won't lie.

I had to meet with nurses, I had to take a sleeping pill I didn't want to take. And I had to stare at 4 white walls.

There was a bunch of chairs and couches in the middle of the room. One lone television blackened, not on, in the midst of it.

At the far end, surrounded by the beautiful view was a kitchen type set-up.

Beyond that was a decrepit looking exercise machine that had been there for however long.

On both sides there were two phones. With lots of information posted all around them.

In among all of this was a dozen or so people. All ages, all races. Some seeming much too young to be on the adult unit (which I later learned was actually from 16 up, not 18) and others seeming dazed to the world around them. I would soon join into the dazed world of life around me.

I drifted back to my room. Plexiglass window in the door, as well as the window, that had another nice view, of a brick wall. Another wing of the hospital.

There was also a stone cold washroom in my room.

In it was a shower, if you could call it that. It didn't stay on. You had to push the button and get water for a couple seconds, over and over again. Didn't think I'd be showering here anyways. Plus, in the cold concrete bathroom, there was no shower curtain, a window in the bathroom door, and best of all no lock. No way was I gonna be stripped naked, freezing my ass off in a shower with minimal privacy at best, in a ward full of "crazy" people.

I went back to my awful little hospital bed and cried. How did it come to this. I needed to talk to my girl. I needed her to know how much I loved her and how sorry I was for all of this. How sorry I was to her, to my children, to my entire world for taking such a drastic escape route.

That though would have to wait till morning as I was not yet allowed to use the phone.

Tears, tears and more tears are what that first night held. I missed my life, my little people and my world. I was so wrong to try to take my life. I still wanted so much to live.

Sylvia Meier

Chapter 4:
So This Is It?!

The first morning was a rough one.

Being awakened by a nurse and told that my breakfast was here and looking around trying to remember where I was when the realization kicks in, oh yeah, here I am, the psych ward.

Stumbling my way to the "kitchen" where all the other inhabitants already sat eating I grabbed the tray with my name and decided I really wasn't hungry. I had barely eaten now in over 24 hours and the appetite just wasn't there. I had no urge to eat, and wanted nothing in my stomach. Most of all, not hospital food. What I really needed was my daily dose of caffeine, but who knew how long it would be till I could have another pepsi.

What I really wanted was to know what exactly the plan of action was and what I had to do to get out of this place. Already I had sensed the real reality sinking in. I was here until they believed me sane and stable enough to leave. One problem... I was unmedicated. If I wasn't stable or even if I was when they brought me in the lack of medication in my system was going to make me unstable very quickly. I could already feel some of the classic symptoms of lithium withdrawal, and was wondering just how bad all of this could get.

I was already starting to feel jittery. This place was more than enough to make me feel uneasy, but the lack of medication was turning me hypo-manic quite quickly.

Before I knew it my name was being called, I was going to be seeing the doc. Oh I'm sure this is going to go just peachy...

In a tiny little room with a couple different doctors we replay the previous night over and over. I express my deep concern at not being medicated. At the fact I knew I needed my medications to remain relatively stable, at the fact I could already feel the energy in my bones. This needed to be put to a halt, but nope, they were gonna give it a day or two, maybe more to decide what I had (What do you mean, what I have, I've HAD bipolar disorder since the day I was born!) and what medication would be right for that.

Ugh.

This was gonna be unpleasant.

To top it off, I was given strict time frames for everything. I could only see those I loved for a few hours here and there, and I was under no circumstances allowed off unit. Looked like I would have to make some friends, or something. This was going to be a really long time here.

And, I was expected to join in on group...

I'm not and never have been one for group settings. Group settings in a psych ward really didn't seem like something I would want to do.

I hoped my girl would come see me that night. I missed her so much. I needed to hold her, to tell her how sorry I was, to make sure she knew this had NOTHING to do with her. And hope that even though this early in our relationship her other half had landed in a psych ward, that she would still love me, and want to be in my life.

I also needed to hear my children's voices. I didn't want them to see me in here. I didn't need that. They were better off simply knowing mommy was in the hospital, not seeing me in this place. At least if I was not to be in here for too long. A week or two maximum was my thoughts. I knew I didn't belong in this place. I simply needed help for a little bit.

I have a hard time socializing under the best of circumstances, add in a lack of medication and an awkward social setting like a psych ward and suddenly I am even worse than ever at meeting anyone. Plus, I wasn't sure I really wanted even causal acquaintances from this place. But being as I had no idea how long I would be here (other than that 5 days was the minimum) I figured better get started. Might make it a little more bearable to be in here.

There weren't that many people to choose from. Two girls who didn't look like they were old enough to be in here, a man with tattoos and a pony-tail. Another one give or take my age and a few others who no longer hold a presence in my mind as I write this.

The blonde girl, maybe 16 seemed safe (minus the mama in me wondering what could she have ever done to land herself in a place like this) so with her I started a casual conversation.

The conversation went on for hours, the guy with the tattoos and pony tail joined us. We had a couple disgusting hospital food meals, I talked to the little ones on the phone, told them how much I missed them already and that mommy was sick and would see them all again soon.

And then finally, my girl walked through the front door.

This was to be the highlight of each day. My girl walking in the door making sure I was alright. Holding me in her arms.

I quickly dragged her out of the main area into my room.

Tears streaked my face, I held her close. I'm sorry, I'm so so sorry. Please, please don't leave me. I was an absolute mess. I loved her so much already and wanted to make sure that even though her girl was locked away, she still wanted me.

She brought me a little teddy bear. His name as I would

determine later would be Lotta Bit bear. My girl always said she loved me lotta bits and so Lotta Bit bear got his name. She loved me lotta bits and Lotta Bit bear would keep me safe in her absence. I clung to her that night. I didn't want her to ever leave. I didn't want to be in here anymore. I wanted to go home. Go home to a home with her, and the kids. I wanted my entire life to change, and I really wanted to live.

It was bittersweet to have her there that night to see me. I was so very happy to see her but so very sad to see her go. I stood there staring at the door as she went through it and I heard the locks clicking into place behind her. What had I really done? What had I done? I loved her so much, already missed her and the children so much my heart ached. This was gonna be a long, long stay.

I went and joined my new "friends" in front of the television. The one hour of television that was allowed had started. After this, it was time for bed. And time for a new day to start.

This time I was given medication to sleep. Perhaps tomorrow they would give me back my medication. Perhaps tomorrow would be better. Called my girl and said good-night. And off to bed I went.

Chapter 5:
The Story Changes...

Time has a tendency to change things, alter your thoughts and make you forget the finer details of the life you had already lived. Medications do the same.

Why, dear reader, you are probably asking is this here in the midst of the story of my time in the psych ward?

Because time and medication, stress and life have done just that.

This book has sat unfinished now staring at me, willing me to finish it and I was unable to. I was unable to gather the thoughts and words that need to fill the blank spaces. I was unable to recall the finer details and that causes major issues when writing a story.

So instead, I offer my sincere apologies for a story half told and will continue this story with what the whole purpose of this particular entry in the "My Bipolar World" series was originially for.

Sylvia Meier

Chapter 6:
Breaking The Stigma

There is such stigma and fear associated with the place in which I found myself in the earlier pages of this story. In the scary, horrifying place called the PYSCH WARD.

You see it on television and it makes it worse. Drooling, scuffling patients without a brain in their head. People who have all but lost their minds, their bodies and their souls to the 4 bare walls.

In reality, it is anything but.

Within those 4 walls yes you may find those in our society who are so far gone that they may never leave those 4 walls, but you also find many others, who like me were simply at the end of a rope and knew no way down. Others who have had things occur in their lives that led them to the safety that is granted by those walls. Men, women and children who are not drooling, lost souls, but vibrant souls begging and pleading with the world to help them get back to the land of the living, to a state of functioning that allows them to resume their lives outside the four walls.

I was scared when I went in, but I was more afraid when I came out.

I knew I was facing the stigma of that place. I knew, being the person that I was, that I wouldn't, couldn't keep my story inside me. I needed to share it with those it could help, those who would listen to the story and perhaps take things away from reading it. I realized as much as I wished no one would know I was in such a place, I would very quickly tell the world I was in such a place and it was not all that the media made it out to be. That it was not at all that which you thought it to be.

Stigma plays a huge role in the our world.

It makes us too quick to judge others. It makes us look at another human and think them to be one way or the other because of something they have.

Mental illness on it's own has a huge stigma attached to it.

In recent years, a lot of more well known people have come out in the public eyes and shared their illness in hope to help destroy the stigma of the illness and show that even people with mental illness are still people. And even with the added difficulties in their lives they are still able to go on and do great things.

Had I believed in the stigma associated with my illness (which for a really long time I did) this book would never have taken shape. I never would have believed I had anything within me worthy of sharing with the world. That I would lack the skills and the mindset to be able to even form the words and type them out.

Had I believed in the stigma of mental illness I would have sat myself on the couch and did nothing with my life, and never would have tried to overcome my illness, even to the levels that I have thus far.

You see a lot of people could have given in to their illnesses and the place would be a much darker world then it is today. Had Beethoven given in to being deaf and decided because he could not hear the music no one would, we would not have his music. Had Stephen Hawking given into his ALS and succumbed to the stigma associated with disabilities we would be without one of the greatest minds of our time. Stephen Fry himself has bipolar disorder and we would be without the humor he injects into the world. And the list goes on.

Had all those who have illnesses and disabilities given into the stigmas that go along with their illness, disabilities or just disabilities in general the world would be a very different place. Even Albert Einstein was thought to have a learning disability!

All of the above names give reason to why we cannot allow stigmas to still exist. All they do is serve to rob us of the potential of the people they are perpetrated upon. They rob us of music, science, and so much more. They need to be put to a stop.

Sylvia Meier

Conclusion:

The biggest thing I want readers to take away from the book in the "My Bipolar World" series is that yes, mental illness is a major condition. Yes, it does bring with it all sorts of issues and problems, but it shouldn't come with stigma. It shouldn't come with pain and heartache simply because of what people traditionally view it as being.

Same holds true with the psych ward. Many of the greatest, most creative individuals in history have been deemed mentally unstable and unfit and spent time in the psych ward.

That doesn't mean they weren't amazing and brilliant. They were nothing of what the stigma holds. They weren't individuals lost in their own world, they weren't shuffling drooling members of society when they were in the psych ward. They were simply the people they are, the brilliant minds they are, needing a little extra help.

Stigma does nothing but destroy those who it is against and disillusion those who believe it. It is a vicious cycle that should not be allowed to continue. I am hoping from reading the words within these pages you realize that not everyone who enters the four walls known as the psych ward is crazy, out of their mind or anything else that is commonly thought. Often they are simply people who need some help to keep their live on track or get back on track.

Sylvia Meier

Other Books By Sylvia Meier

Living Bipolar: Learning To Live With Bipolar Disorder

http://www.amazon.com/Living-Bipolar-My-World-ebook/dp/B00CP58BLI/

http://www.amazon.com/Living-Bipolar-Learning-Live-Disorder/dp/1484816366/

Bipolar Bits: Manic Madness To Depressive Depths

http://www.amazon.com/Bipolar-Bits-Madness-Depressive-ebook/dp/B00CW667IY/

http://www.amazon.com/Bipolar-Bits-Madness-Depressive-Depths/dp/1484990722/

Lotta Bipolar Bits: Survivors Diary Of Living Bipolar

http://www.amazon.com/Lotta-Bipolar-Bits-Survivors-ebook/dp/B00D2VZ3TW/

http://www.amazon.com/Lotta-Bipolar-Bits-Survivors-Living/dp/1489589368/

My Bipolar World: A Collection Of Works By Sylvia Meier

http://www.amazon.com/My-Bipolar-World-Collection-ebook/dp/B00D2XY8QO/

http://www.amazon.com/My-Bipolar-World-Collection-Sylvia/dp/1489517030

Bipolar Hope: Discovering Hope In Your Diagnosis

http://www.amazon.com/Bipolar-Hope-Discovering-Diagnosis-ebook/dp/B00D9WSLUC

http://www.amazon.com/Bipolar-Hope-Discovering-Diagnosis-World/dp/1490370706

Relapse, Remission and Stability: The 3 Stages Of Bipolar Disorder

http://www.amazon.com/Relapse-Remission-Stability-Bipolar-ebook/dp/B00DOJIET8

http://www.amazon.com/Relapse-Remission-Stability-Bipolar-Disorder/dp/1490370668

7

COMING SOON:

- **My Bipolar World: A Second Collection Of Works By Sylvia Meier**

- **Support And Bipolar: You Need More Than Just You**

- **The Claws And Embrace: Depression In Bipolar Disorder**

- **Manic, Misery And More: The Upswing Of Living Bipolar**

- **My Bipolar World: A Third Collection Of Works By Sylvia Meier**

Sylvia Meier

ABOUT THE AUTHOR

I'm not doing this about the author is traditional fashion. It's awkward and plain strange to write about myself in the third person.

My name is Sylvia.

I'll be 32 this summer.

I am the mother of 5 beautiful children.

I am the partner of the beautiful woman who has been my greatest support in my fight.

I am living bipolar. I have bipolar disorder type one. I was first diagnosed at 13 years old, and went through the typical denial and rebellion.

Fast forward 17 years and life is off-kilter, all sorts of wrong, my illness has left my life shattered, tattered and my life on a string.

Suicide attempt, stopped by myself was the best and worst moment of my life. It was the wake up call I needed, and the scare I needed. I took my illness in my hands, decided to be in control instead of my disorder being in control and here I am a year later in the best mental health of my life.

I won't lie, there are days that are tough, there are days I long to be manic again. Overall though, I am happy, I am healthy and I have more support in my life than I could ever imagine.

I am a writer by passion. This is not my first book and surely will not be my last. I am in the process of writing another one called "Woman Broken, A Child Lost" which is about my life, my struggles and everything in between. It too will hopefully be out this year, but is one of those stories that will not be released until perfection is reached as it is my story. My full story.

Till then you can always find me and support for yourself on my website which is my story and writings as well. Check it out at http://www.MyBipolarWorld.com

In the end, I send you all much love and hope. If you take nothing else from all of this at least know you are not alone, and if you ever need that ear, feel free to contact me at my site. I do my best to respond to everyone as time and living bipolar allows.

Love,
  Sylvia